AMANDA WOOD

A journey to natural wellness

a semi-crunchy mom's beginner's guide

The information provided in this book should not be used for diagnosing or treating a health problem or disease, and those seeking personal medical advice should consult with a licensed physician. Always seek the advice of your doctor or other qualified health provider regarding a medical condition.

First edition

This book was professionally typeset on Reedsy.
Find out more at reedsy.com

Contents

Introduction 1

Chapter 1 : What, where & why of toxins 4

Chapter 2 : Nurturing Women's Wellness 8

Chapter 3 : Essential oils 11

Chapter 4 : Simple swaps 28

Chapter 5: Closing thoughts 32

About the Author 33

Introduction

Welcome to the enchanting realm of natural and holistic wellness, where nature's treasures hold the power to transform your well-being. In a world filled with hustle and bustle, it's easy to overlook the subtle impact our daily choices have on our well-being.

This book aims to guide you through the transformative process of reevaluating the products you use, the food you consume, and the environment you create within your home. As we embark on this exploration together, we'll unravel the layers of toxicity that can unknowingly infiltrate our lives. From household cleaners to personal care products, we'll examine the hidden chemicals that may compromise our health and the planet. But fear not, for this journey is not about sacrifice; it's about making informed choices that enhance our lives and the world around us.

Through the pages that follow, we'll delve into the principles of non-toxic living, offering practical tips, actionable steps, and insights into the positive impact these changes can have on your overall well-being. Join me in embracing a lifestyle that not only nurtures your body but also fosters a sustainable and thriving world for generations to come.

In this introductory chapter, I will share a little bit about myself and how I got started on my own journey. My hope is that in sharing my journey it will encourage you to make some simple lifestyle switches for your generations to come.

My name is Amanda Wood and I am a wife & mother who lives in the backwoods of nowhere Georgia. Seven years ago we lived right outside the city living basically the same life everyone else was living. I bought all of our cleaning and bath products at the store and didn't think anything about it. At the time I had a 2 year-old daughter who was struggling with ear infections. The doctors couldn't find an antibiotic that could clear up the infection and at this point she had infection coming out of her ear. We had already been through one set of tubes and were having to go back in for another set. Then my cousin introduced me to essential oils. They were my gateway into natural and holistic wellness. I started applying tea tree, lavender & frankincense to the bottoms of her feet morning and night. When we went in for our tubal surgery the doctor told us that her infection had completely cleared up.

HUGE DISCLAIMER! I am not a doctor. I am not offering cures or remedies. I'm only sharing my experiences with recipes that I will share at the end of this book.

After my daughter's surgery I jumped into the essential oil community on social media and my eyes were open to the hazards in our environment, but most surprising was how it was affecting our bodies. Do you struggle with fatigue, headaches, skin issues, loss of hair, brain fog, moodiness, heavy or painful periods? Your environment or the things you put on or in your body could be a contributing factor to these things or more. Please hear me when I say I do not say these things to scare you, but to make you aware so that you can make some changes to possibly get relief. Let's get started.

Chapter 1 : What, where & why of toxins

I know I've talked a lot about hazards in your environment, but what are they and where can we find them? In our pursuit of convenience and cleanliness, we can unknowingly expose ourselves to a multitude of hidden dangers. This chapter sheds light on the potential hazards posed by common household chemicals. Before we dive in though, remember we will not be able to avoid all toxins around us. So please give yourself grace. This book is meant to bring awareness not shame. You cannot change what has been done, but you can change for what is to come.

Cleaning Products:

Most of your common cleaning products purchased at the store often contain volatile organic compounds (VOCs) that can contribute to indoor air pollution. Long-term exposure may lead to respiratory issues, headaches, and other health concerns. Opting for eco-friendly alternatives can mitigate these risks.

Fragrance:

Fragrances in air fresheners and cleaning products may contain phthalates, linked to hormonal disruptions. Choosing fragrance-free options can help minimize the impact on your health and that of your family. Candles are another hazard. Burning a candle for one hour is the equivalent to smoking a cigarette in your home.

Pesticides:

Pesticides, although effective in controlling pests, can be harmful to humans. Prolonged exposure may contribute to neurological issues and respiratory complications. Integrated pest management and natural repellents offer safer alternatives.

Cookware:

Certain cookware, like nonstick pans, may release harmful chemicals when heated. Choosing stainless steel, cast iron, or ceramic alternatives can reduce the risk of chemical exposure during food preparation.

Plastics:

Plastic containers, especially those with BPA, may leach harmful chemicals into food and beverages. Opting for glass or BPA-free plastics ensures a safer choice for storing and consuming edibles.

Laundry Room:

Laundry detergents and fabric softeners may contain chemicals that can irritate the skin and cause respiratory distress. Switching to fragrance-free and hypoallergenic options or even making your own can help mitigate these risks.

Conclusion:

While it's convenient to buy household products from the store and bring them into our homes, understanding the potential dangers they pose is paramount. By making informed choices and opting for safer alternatives, we can create a home environment that promotes well-being and longevity. The path to a healthier home starts with awareness and a commitment to reducing exposure to harmful chemicals.

Chapter 2 : Nurturing Women's Wellness

One of the hidden dangers of toxins that shocked me was affecting my reproductive system. When I learned what I will be sharing with you I knew I had to do better for my daughter. She deserved a better start than me. Being aware of the impact of environmental toxins on reproductive health is crucial. From endocrine disruptors to pollutants, awareness empowers women to make informed choices, fostering a healthier environment for themselves and future generations. This chapter explores the relationship between reproductive health and embracing a toxin-free lifestyle.

The Menstrual Cycle:

The menstrual cycle is a complex and intricate biological process that plays a crucial role in the reproductive health of women. However, amidst the marvel of this monthly occurrence, it is essential to understand the potential risks associated with toxin exposure during this time. The menstrual cycle consists of several phases, including menstruation, the follicular phase, ovulation, and the luteal phase. Each phase is regulated by hormonal fluctuations, primarily estrogen and progesterone. This intricate dance of hormones orchestrates the shedding of the uterine lining, the release of an egg, and the preparation of the body for a potential pregnancy.

Toxins effect on menstrual cycle:

Toxins present in our environment, often referred to as endocrine-disrupting chemicals (EDCs), can interfere with the delicate hormonal balance of the menstrual cycle. Common toxins include pesticides, heavy metals, and certain plastics. These substances can mimic or block hormones, leading to irregularities in the menstrual cycle, delayed ovulation, and even fertility issues. Surprisingly, some menstrual products may contribute to toxin exposure. Certain sanitary pads and tampons can contain trace amounts of harmful substances, such as dioxins and synthetic fragrances. While these levels are generally considered low and within safety limits, long-term and cumulative exposure remains a concern. Opt for organic tampons and pads to reduce the risk of exposure to pesticides and other harmful chemicals. Silicone or latex menstrual cups are reusable and can be a safer alternative to disposable products, minimizing environmental impact and potential toxin exposure.

Personal care products:

The Environmental Working Group Survey found that on average, American women put 168 chemicals on their bodies each day... The group found that chemicals from the products used were ending up inside their bodies. It's important to evaluate the ingredients in your personal care products, including soaps and lotions, as some may contain EDCs that could impact hormonal health. Understanding the interplay between the menstrual cycle and toxin hazards is vital for promoting reproductive well-being. By making informed choices about menstrual products and adopting a conscious lifestyle, you can take proactive steps to minimize toxin exposure and support a healthy menstrual cycle.

Chapter 3 : Essential oils

Essential oils are what started me on this journey and what I turn to quite often. In this chapter we embark on a journey into the heart of aromatherapy, unraveling the mysteries of essential oils for beginners. From their ancient origins to the modern resurgence of interest, we'll explore the diverse and therapeutic possibilities these precious oils offer. The reason I'm going into so much detail on essential oils is because you can do so many simple swaps in your home with them. Essential oils, often distilled through methods like steam distillation or cold pressing, contain the essence and fragrance of the source plant. Each essential oil boasts a unique composition, contributing to its distinct properties and potential health benefits.

What are essential oils and where did they come from? Essential oils are concentrated hydrophobic liquids containing volatile aroma compounds from plants. These compounds are responsible for the characteristic fragrance and therapeutic qualities associated with essential oils. Extracted from different parts of plants such as leaves, flowers, bark, or roots, these oils have been used for centuries in various cultures for their medicinal, cosmetic, and even spiritual purposes. The chemical composition of essential oils is intricate, with each oil comprising a blend of compounds such as terpenes, phenols, aldehydes, and esters. It's this intricate mix that gives each essential oil its unique scent and therapeutic effects. For example, lavender essential oil is renowned for its calming properties, while lemongrass oil is celebrated for its antimicrobial prowess.

One of the significant roles of essential oils is their use in aromatherapy. The inhalation of these aromatic compounds is believed to stimulate brain function, influencing emotions and mood. Lavender and citrus oils are often used to promote relaxation, alleviate stress, and improve overall emotional well-being. Beyond their aromatic influence, essential oils are celebrated for their potential health benefits. Some essential oils, like eucalyptus and peppermint, are recognized for their respiratory benefits, helping to clear congestion. Tea tree oil is known for its antimicrobial properties, making it a popular choice for skin issues.

Essential oils can be applied in various ways, including aromatherapy diffusers, topical application (when diluted with carrier oils), and even ingested under the guidance of a qualified professional. It's essential to note that while essential oils offer a range of potential benefits, they should be used with caution, as concentrated forms may cause irritation or adverse reactions in certain individuals. Ensuring the quality and purity of essential oils is paramount. With an influx of products in the market, it's crucial to source oils from reputable suppliers to guarantee authenticity and avoid adulteration. Pure essential oils retain the full spectrum of therapeutic compounds, maximizing their potential benefits.

The roots of essential oils can be traced to ancient civilizations where plants were revered not only for sustenance but also for their perceived healing properties. In Egypt, hieroglyphics and papyrus scrolls reveal the use of essential oils in embalming practices and rituals. The aromatic essences were associated with purification and offerings to deities.

The ancient Greeks expanded the understanding of botanical extracts. The physician Hippocrates, often regarded as the father of medicine, recognized the medicinal properties of aromatic plants. Likewise, the Romans utilized essential oils for perfumes, cosmetics, and therapeutic purposes. The famous physician Galen further contributed to the knowledge of plant extracts in medical practices. During the Middle Ages, the knowledge of essential oils endured through the Islamic Golden Age.

Scholars translated Greek and Roman texts, preserving and augmenting the understanding of aromatics. Avicenna, an influential Persian polymath, documented essential oil distillation methods in the 11th century, laying the groundwork for future advancements. The Renaissance era witnessed a resurgence of interest in herbalism and natural remedies. Essential oils became integral to the practices of herbalists and alchemists. Notably, Paracelsus, a Swiss-German physician, emphasized the healing properties of plants, contributing to the evolving field of aromatherapy.

The 19th century marked a pivotal period for essential oils. The advent of steam distillation in the early 1800s revolutionized the extraction process, making it more efficient and accessible.

Renowned figures like Madame Maury and René-Maurice Gatte-fossé began exploring the therapeutic applications of essential oils, laying the foundation for modern aromatherapy.

The 20th century witnessed a resurgence of interest in natural remedies and alternative medicine. The term "aromatherapy" was coined by René-Maurice Gattefossé in the 1920s, signifying the therapeutic use of essential oils. Influential personalities like Marguerite Maury and Jean Valnet further popularized aromatherapy, contributing to its integration into mainstream wellness practices.

In the present day, essential oils have become ingrained in diverse cultures and practices worldwide. Their popularity extends beyond alternative medicine, with applications in skin-care, stress relief, and even household cleaning products. On-going scientific research continues to explore the efficacy and safety of essential oils, ensuring their place in the evolving landscape of holistic health.

Enough history and science now I will talk about the 10 essential oils that are most used in our home. Some of the following information might sound a little scientific, but tick with me.

Peppermint

Comes from the leaves of the peppermint plant (Mentha × piperita), this oil boasts a myriad of benefits. Peppermint's invigorating scent has the power to awaken the senses. Diffusing a few drops can promote mental clarity and provide a burst of energy, making it a popular choice for home and office environments. Known for its cooling properties, peppermint essential oil is a go-to for soothing various discomforts. I like to put it on the back of my neck for a quick cool down in the middle of summer. Diluted and applied topically, it can alleviate tension and promote a calming sensation on muscles and joints. Peppermint has a long history of being used to support respiratory health. Inhaling its vapor can help clear nasal passages, making it a trusted ally during seasonal challenges or times of congestion. I've actually seen oxygen numbers increase when peppermint oil is around. Aiding digestion is among peppermint's digestive benefits.

Whether ingested in a diluted form or added to tea, it can provide relief from occasional indigestion and support a healthy digestive system. The strong aroma of peppermint is a natural deterrent for pests. Spritzing a diluted solution around your home or garden can help keep unwanted visitors at bay without resorting to harsh chemicals. Peppermint's invigorating aroma isn't just a treat for the nose; it can also enhance focus and concentration. Inhaling the scent while working or studying may contribute to heightened cognitive performance.

While peppermint oil offers a multitude of benefits, it's essential to use it with care. Peppermint oil is considered a hot oil, which means when used topically you will feel a sensation on the skin. Due to its potency, it's advisable to dilute before applying topically and consult with a healthcare professional, especially for those with sensitive skin or medical conditions. As with any essential oil, quality matters. Seek out reputable sources to ensure purity and potency.

Lavender

Lavandula angustifolia, commonly known as true lavender, is the primary source of lavender essential oil. Native to the Mediterranean region, this hardy, woody shrub boasts slender spikes of vibrant purple flowers that exude a captivating scent. Lavender essential oil is typically extracted through steam distillation, preserving its aromatic and therapeutic properties. The oil's composition includes compounds like linalool and linalyl acetate, contributing to its distinct floral and herbaceous fragrance.

Lavender's soothing aroma is renowned for its calming effects on the mind and body. Used in aromatherapy, the oil helps alleviate stress, anxiety, and promotes relaxation. A few drops in a diffuser can transform any space into a haven of tranquility. Lavender's sedative qualities make it a popular choice for improving sleep quality. Incorporating lavender oil into a bedtime routine, whether through diffusing or adding a drop to a pillow, can promote a restful night's sleep. Lavender's gentle nature extends to skincare, where it proves beneficial for various skin conditions.

Its anti-inflammatory and antimicrobial properties make it a valuable addition to creams, lotions, and even DIY face masks, helping to soothe irritated skin. I make sure to have it on hand in the kitchen in case of burns. Lavender's natural insect-repelling properties make it an eco-friendly alternative to chemical-laden repellents. A diluted solution can be applied to the skin or infused in candles to ward off unwanted pests.

While lavender is generally considered safe for most individuals, some may experience skin irritation. Always perform a patch test and consult with a healthcare professional, especially for pregnant women or those with pre-existing conditions.

Lemon

Extracted from the Citrus limon plant, this golden elixir has graced kitchens, apothecaries, and aromatherapy sessions for centuries. Lemon essential oil is a symphony of citrus notes, awakening the senses with its crisp, clean fragrance. Its lively aroma has the power to uplift moods and create a refreshing ambiance, making it a staple in aromatherapy practices. Whether diffused, inhaled, or applied topically, the oil's aromatic influence can evoke a sense of clarity and positivity.

Beyond its aromatic appeal, lemon essential oil boasts potent cleansing properties. Its high concentration of limonene, a natural compound found in citrus fruits, makes it a formidable ally in household cleaning. From surfaces to air, this oil acts as a natural purifier, leaving behind a pristine environment. I've used it to remove stickers and hard to remove bandages too. Rich in vitamin C, lemon essential oil offers more than just a delightful scent.

When used topically, it can support skin health, promoting a radiant complexion. Its astringent properties make it a popular choice for those seeking to tone and rejuvenate their skin. Lemon essential oil isn't confined to the realm of wellness; it also makes a noteworthy appearance in culinary pursuits. A drop or two can transform dishes, imparting a burst of citrus flavor without the need for squeezing lemons. From desserts to savory dishes, this oil adds a zesty twist to culinary creations.

While lemon is considered safe it is a photosensitive oil and will cause dark spots on the skin if exposed to light.

Eucalyptus

Derived from the leaves of the eucalyptus tree, this essential oil has been cherished for centuries, celebrated for its healing properties and aromatic allure. The eucalyptus tree, native to Australia, serves as the primary source of eucalyptus essential oil. With over 700 species, the most commonly used are Eucalyptus globulus and Eucalyptus radiata. Recognizable by its tall stature and distinctive, aromatic leaves, the eucalyptus tree has become an emblem of vitality and resilience.

Eucalyptus essential oil is renowned for its respiratory benefits. Inhalation of its invigorating scent can open airways, making it a popular choice for addressing congestion and respiratory issues. The oil's active compound, cineole, has been shown to have antiviral and antimicrobial properties, enhancing its efficacy in promoting respiratory health.

Beyond its respiratory advantages, eucalyptus oil is a stalwart defender of the immune system. Its antibacterial properties contribute to its role in fighting infections, while its anti-inflammatory nature aids in reducing inflammation, promoting a quicker recovery from various ailments. Eucalyptus essential oil isn't limited to physical wellness; it also has a soothing effect on the mind. Its refreshing aroma can alleviate mental fatigue, promote mental clarity, and invigorate the senses. Diffusing eucalyptus oil in spaces where concentration is key, such as offices or study areas, can enhance cognitive performance.

Diluted eucalyptus oil can be applied topically for skin-related concerns, offering relief from insect bites, minor wounds, and skin irritations. It's important, however, to heed proper dilution ratios and conduct a patch test to ensure compatibility with individual skin types. Eucalyptus oil's versatile aroma pairs well with various essential oils. Combining it with peppermint creates a helpful respiratory blend, while blending it with lavender introduces a calming element for mind and sore muscles if added to a bath with epsom salts.

Though eucalyptus is generally safe, caution is advised, especially for those with respiratory conditions, young children, or pregnant individuals. Always consult with a healthcare professional before incorporating eucalyptus oil into wellness routines.

Tea tree

Tea tree oil is derived from the leaves of the Melaleuca alternifolia tree, a species native to the northeastern coast of Australia. Indigenous Australian communities have long recognized the medicinal value of the tea tree, using its leaves to treat wounds, infections, and various skin ailments. The potency of tea tree oil lies in its complex composition. Rich in terpenes, particularly terpinen-4-ol, cineole, and alpha-terpinene, it exhibits remarkable antimicrobial and anti-inflammatory properties. These compounds contribute to the oil's effectiveness in combating bacteria, viruses, and fungi.

Tea tree oil's reputation as a natural antimicrobial agent is well-founded. Studies have highlighted its efficacy against a wide spectrum of microorganisms, making it a popular choice for treating skin infections, cuts, and even acne. Its ability to inhibit the growth of bacteria and fungi has positioned it as a valuable tool in natural skincare.

Beyond its antimicrobial prowess, tea tree oil is renowned for its ability to soothe various skin conditions. Whether addressing irritation, itching, or inflammation, its anti-inflammatory properties make it a go-to remedy for conditions like eczema, psoriasis, and dermatitis. When inhaled, its vapors can help alleviate respiratory issues. Its expectorant properties make it useful in easing congestion and coughs, providing a natural alternative for respiratory support.

Tea tree oil can be applied topically when diluted with a carrier oil to prevent skin irritation. It is commonly found in skincare products such as creams, lotions, and shampoos. Additionally, its aromatic qualities make it suitable for diffusion in aromatherapy practices. As with any essential oil, a patch test is recommended, especially for those with sensitive skin.

Ylang ylang

Native to the tropical rainforests of countries like Indonesia, Malaysia, and the Philippines, the ylang-ylang tree produces star-shaped, yellow flowers. Cultivated for centuries, these blossoms are meticulously harvested to extract the precious essential oil, renowned for its captivating aroma and therapeutic benefits. Ylang-ylang essential oil is obtained through steam distillation of the freshly picked flowers. The distillation process is conducted with precision to capture the intricate layers of fragrance, resulting in multiple grades of oil – Extra, Grade I, Grade II, and Grade III. Each grade possesses a unique aroma profile, ranging from intensely floral to subtly sweet.

Ylang-ylang's scent is a symphony of floral, fruity, and slightly spicy notes. The oil is cherished for its ability to soothe the mind and evoke feelings of joy. Its complex aroma is often used in perfumery, where it serves as a heart note, blending harmoniously with other essential oils to create captivating fragrances. Beyond its captivating fragrance, ylang-ylang essential oil is revered for its therapeutic properties. Known for its calming effects, it is frequently used in aromatherapy to alleviate stress, anxiety, and tension. The oil is believed to promote emotional balance, making it a valuable tool for relaxation and promoting a positive mindset.

Ylang-ylang's benefits extend beyond aromatherapy. In skincare, it is utilized for its hydrating properties and ability to balance sebum production, making it suitable for both dry and oily skin types. The oil is also employed in hair care products, contributing to the health and shine of the hair. The oil is used in massage blends, diffusers, and baths, creating an atmosphere of serenity and relaxation. While ylang-ylang essential oil offers a multitude of benefits, some individuals may be sensitive to its strong aroma, and excessive use can lead to headaches or nausea. Dilution and moderation are key when incorporating ylang-ylang into personal care or wellness routines.

Lemongrass

Derived from the tall, thin blades of the Cymbopogon citratus plant, lemongrass essential oil has captured the hearts of aromatherapy enthusiasts and holistic health practitioners alike. Lemongrass, native to tropical regions like Southeast Asia and Africa, has a long history of traditional medicinal use. Cultivated for its flavorful culinary contributions and therapeutic properties, this grassy plant has become synonymous with freshness and vitality.

The unmistakable citrusy and lemony fragrance of lemongrass is renowned for its ability to uplift moods, promote mental clarity, and dispel feelings of lethargy. Diffusing lemongrass oil in your living space can transform it into a sanctuary of positivity. Lemongrass oil is celebrated for its antimicrobial and antifungal properties. When diffused or applied topically, it serves as a natural purifier, creating an environment that discourages unwanted microbes.

Its astringent properties make it a popular choice in skincare routines. Diluted lemongrass oil can be applied to the skin, helping to tone and rejuvenate, while also addressing issues like acne and oily skin. Lemongrass essential oil is often incorporated into massage blends for its potential to soothe muscle aches and joint discomfort. Its analgesic properties offer a natural solution for those seeking relief from physical tension.

Beyond its aromatic and therapeutic attributes, lemongrass is a culinary gem. Widely used in Asian cuisine, it adds a citrusy zing to soups, curries, and marinades. Extracting the essential oil allows chefs and home cooks to infuse dishes with the distinct flavor of lemongrass.

Lemongrass oil's insect-repelling properties make it a popular choice for creating natural bug sprays. Its refreshing scent acts as a deterrent while keeping outdoor activities enjoyable. Inhaling lemongrass oil can provide a quick and effective way to alleviate stress and tension. A few drops in a diffuser or added to a warm bath can create a serene atmosphere.

Always dilute the oil before applying it to the skin, and perform a patch test to check for sensitivities. Pregnant individuals and those with certain medical conditions should consult with a healthcare professional before using lemongrass oil.

Clove

Derived from the Syzygium aromaticum tree's dried flower buds, this aromatic elixir has woven its fragrant tapestry through centuries of human history. Clove, with its origins in the Maluku Islands of Indonesia, has been revered for its culinary and medicinal properties for over 2,000 years. Traders and explorers coveted cloves, and the spice became a symbol of wealth and prestige. The extraction process of clove essential oil is an intricate dance between art and science. The unopened flower buds are carefully harvested by hand just before they bloom, ensuring the highest concentration of aromatic compounds. Steam distillation then captures the essence, producing a potent oil that embodies the warm, spicy, and slightly fruity aroma of cloves.

In traditional medicine, clove oil has been a trusted remedy for various ailments. Its natural antiseptic and analgesic properties have made it a staple in oral care, easing toothaches and promoting overall dental health. Clove essential oil is a treasure trove of therapeutic benefits. Its chief component, eugenol, exhibits potent antioxidant and anti-inflammatory properties. This makes clove oil a valuable asset in supporting the body's natural defenses against oxidative stress and inflammation.

In aromatherapy, the scent of clove oil is hailed for its ability to evoke a sense of warmth and comfort. Diffusing this oil can create an inviting ambiance, promoting relaxation and mental well-being. Beyond its aromatic allure, clove oil showcases remarkable versatility. It is a popular ingredient in skincare, known for its ability to promote a clear complexion and soothe skin irritations. Diluted clove oil can be applied topically to alleviate muscle and joint discomfort, offering natural relief.

Clove oil is considered a hot oil, which means when used topically you will feel a sensation on the skin. Due to its concentrated nature, dilution is key to prevent skin irritation. Pregnant individuals and young children should exercise caution, and consulting with a healthcare professional is advised before incorporating clove oil into any wellness routine.

Rosemary

Native to the Mediterranean region, the herbaceous rosemary plant (Rosmarinus officinalis) has a rich history dating back centuries. Revered by ancient cultures for its aromatic allure and medicinal properties, rosemary's essence has been captured through meticulous extraction processes to create the prized essential oil we cherish today. The process of extracting rosemary essential oil is an art, involving the steam distillation of the plant's flowering tops. This gentle method ensures that the volatile compounds responsible for the oil's distinctive fragrance and therapeutic effects are carefully preserved. The result is a concentrated elixir that embodies the essence of the herb in its purest form.

Rosemary essential oil is celebrated for its invigorating scent, known to stimulate the senses and enhance mental clarity. Diffusing this aromatic oil can create an uplifting atmosphere, making it a popular choice for those seeking focus and concentration during work or study. Beyond its aromatic charm, rosemary essential oil boasts a myriad of health benefits. Rich in antioxidants and antimicrobial properties, it has been used traditionally to support respiratory health, ease muscle tension, and promote overall well-being. Incorporating rosemary oil into massage blends or topical applications can provide a soothing and rejuvenating experience.

Rosemary transcends its traditional uses and finds a place in culinary pursuits. A drop or two of high-quality rosemary essential oil can impart a delightful flavor to dishes, adding a fragrant touch to both savory and sweet creations. From roasted vegetables to baked goods, its culinary versatility is a testament to its enduring appeal. The nourishing properties of rosemary essential oil extend to skincare, where it is embraced for its ability to promote a healthy complexion. Whether blended into skincare products or added to homemade masks and serums, rosemary oil contributes to a radiant and refreshed appearance.

Thyme

Derived from the perennial herb Thymus vulgaris, thyme essential oil has been celebrated for its therapeutic properties throughout history. Thyme, a member of the mint family, is native to the Mediterranean region. Its tiny purple flowers give way to the extraction of the essential oil through steam distillation. This meticulous process captures the essence of thyme, resulting in a potent and concentrated oil.

The fragrance of thyme essential oil is invigorating and herbaceous, making it a popular choice in aromatherapy. Its warm and comforting aroma has been known to elevate mood, reduce stress, and promote mental clarity. Diffusing thyme oil creates an ambiance that revitalizes both mind and spirit.

Thyme has been revered for its antimicrobial properties since ancient times. The essential oil contains compounds like thymol, known for their ability to combat bacteria and fungi. Thyme oil's antimicrobial prowess makes it a natural choice for disinfecting surfaces and supporting the immune system. Inhaling thyme essential oil can be a breath of fresh air for respiratory health. Its expectorant properties may help alleviate coughs and congestion. Incorporating thyme oil into steam inhalation or adding a few drops to a diffuser during the cold season can provide relief and promote easier breathing.

Thyme essential oil is a potent ally in skincare. Its antiseptic and anti-inflammatory properties make it a valuable addition to topical applications. Diluted with a carrier oil, thyme oil can be applied to minor skin irritations, helping to soothe and support the healing process.

Beyond its therapeutic benefits, thyme has made its mark in the culinary world. Widely used in Mediterranean cuisine, this herb imparts a savory and earthy flavor to dishes. Thyme essential oil, when used sparingly, can enhance the taste of soups, stews, and various culinary creations. While thyme essential oil offers numerous benefits, it should be used with care. Due to its potency, it's recommended to dilute it before topical application and be mindful of potential skin sensitivity.

Chapter 4 : Simple swaps

One of the first things I did after learning about the dangers of store bought cleaners and bath products was start switching them out for natural alternatives. DISCLAIMER: I haven't switched everything out and I didn't switch everything out in one fell swoop. It took time, so please give yourself time and grace. Here are some simple switches you can make through alternative purchase or DIY.

Household cleaner:

An alternative I use is Revive Immune Boosting cleaner. It's an easy swap for our family that keeps the house clean and the air even cleaner. I simply purchased a 32 oz spray bottle and added a capful of the concentrated cleaner and filled the rest of it up with water.

A DIY alternative would be to fill a spray bottle halfway with vinegar or alcohol. Add 10-15 drops of clove & lemon essential oils, which can be purchased through many online companies, and fill the rest of the bottle up with water.

Room spray:

An alternative I use is to make my own sprays or purchase safe sprays from companies I've done research to make sure there aren't any harmful chemicals.

A DIY alternative is to fill a small spray bottle halfway with witch hazel and add 10-15 drops of your favorite essential oils. I like a blend of geranium & lemon. Just fill the bottle the rest of the way with water and spray away!

Bath products:

Navigating the labyrinth of personal care products, cosmetics, and household items can be daunting. Discovering toxin-free alternatives ensures that you are not unwittingly exposing your family to harmful substances and safeguarding reproductive well-being. Your best friend in the bathroom is going to be Castile soap, if you are making your own bath products like, body wash, face wash & hand soap. I'm using Dr. Natural right now, but you find what is best for you and your family. There are many good companies that make the swap a one stop shop. I encourage you to find something like that to help make this transition easier.

If you want to start with a simple DIY that can be used as a body & face wash & hand soap I get an empty 8-12 oz foaming pump bottle. I put ¼ cup of castor oil, ½ cup castile soap & 10-15 drops of your favorite essential oils. I then fill the bottle with water, shake, and use it as needed.

Laundry soap:

Again there are many clean companies that offer subscriptions for household items, including laundry soap, dish soap & even dishwasher detergent. It's definitely an easy button to swap your home to a toxin free environment. If you're like me though I like to make things. Here is a recipe I use for laundry soap.

First, heat up 2 gallons of water on the stove. Next, grate a 2 bars of castile soap of your choice with a box grater or food processor. I prefer to use my food processor to really speed the process up. Add the grated soap to the hot, but not boiling water and remove from heat. Stir until soap is dissolved. Next, measure out 3 cups of Arm & Hammer Baking Soda, 3 cups of borax and 3 cups of Arm & Hammer super washing soda and add them to the hot water mixture. Add 1/2 gallon of water to a 5-gallon bucket. Stir in the hot water mixture and stir often. Add 30 to 50 drops of the essential oil of choice. Fill the bucket the rest of the way with water. Stir until all ingredients are well combined. Let it sit overnight and then shake the bucket really well.

NOTES: I like to pour the detergent in a 1/2 gallon jar to make use easier. You can also store it in old laundry soap containers. Shake well before each use. Use 1/2 cup of detergent per load.

Chapter 5: Closing thoughts

I really appreciate you reading this beginner's guide to non-toxic living. I also appreciate someone who is passionate about keeping their family safe. We have the power to give our children a healthier start than what society is pushing. I got a lot of eye rolls at first, but COVID changed that. People slowed down and realized maybe we needed to make some changes and ask some questions. I really encourage you to let this book be a beginning. There is so much information out there and I'm still learning daily. Like I said before I know that we cannot escape all toxins in our environment, but the simple swaps I have done have made a huge difference in my family's health. Thank you again and good luck in your journey.

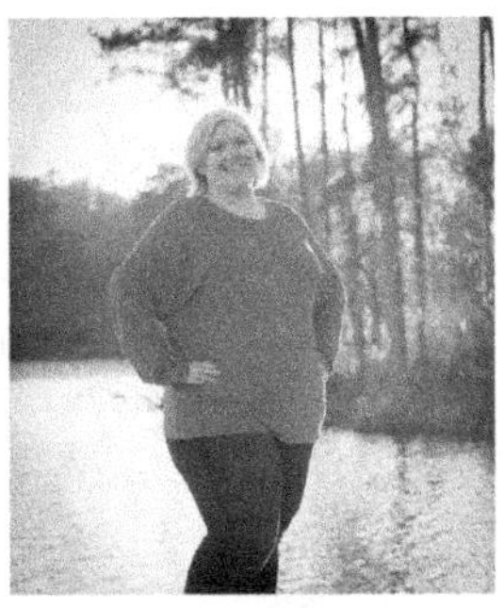

About the Author

Amanda Wood is a Christian Life coach that became interested in holistic living in 2017. *A journey to natural wellness* is her debut book and the beginning of her journey to putting her knowledge into print. She lives in Georgia with her husband, son & daughter. Find her on TikTok.

www.ingramcontent.com/pod-product-compliance
Lightning Source LLC
Chambersburg PA
CBHW050753250726
48662CB00005B/2202